# THE IMPACT OF DIGITAL TECHNOLOGY ON CHILDHOOD ANXIETY

# THE IMPACT OF DIGITAL TECHNOLOGY ON CHILDHOOD ANXIETY

GRETA ROSE

# CONTENTS

Introduction   1

**1** Understanding Childhood Anxiety   5

**2** The Digital Age: A New Frontier for Childhood Deve   11

**3** The Intersection of Digital Technology and Childho   15

**4** Parenting in the Digital Age   19

**5** Schools and Mental Health Support   23

**6** Future Directions for Research and Policy   27

**7** Conclusion   31

Copyright © 2024 by Greta Rose
All rights reserved. No part of this book may be reproduced in any manner whatsoever without written permission except in the case of brief quotations embodied in critical articles and reviews.
First Printing, 2024

# Introduction

Consider for a minute an average child. Try to take a mental note of their environment. Chances are, the digital world will be drawing them in more than any other element in their surroundings. For many children under the age of 8, digital devices have always existed as part of their everyday life. They see their parents constantly holding mobile phones, cannot recall a world without high definition gaming graphics, and regularly engage in swapping Pokemon around the world on their gaming devices. Embedded within today's digital age, platforms like YouTube or TikTok have greatly influenced the unfolding of children's play, access to consumer culture, and cultivation of social chains around the globe. Arguably, digital technology has radically reshaped our society and transformed the very way children think, learn, and engage with others.

Furthermore, children's elevated reliance on digital screen time and gaming has fueled serious debates and concerns amongst scholars, practitioners, and the general public that have escalated in recent years. The extensive use of digital devices for pleasure activities is closely associated with a kaleidoscope of adverse health outcomes, including disturbances in circadian rhythms, obesity, disrupted neuro-development, and increased rates of sedentary behavior-associated disorders. Recent research has imposed a particular emphasis on examining the negative psychological outcomes of adopting digital technology, given children's underdeveloped cognitive ability. Of all the psychological disturbances, a persistent mental health problem lacks the attention and investment it so desperately requires – namely, childhood anxiety.

*Background and Rationale*

The development of duty of care and the fragmentation of childhood; recent national studies into the mental health of Kiwi children aged 2 to 19 years organization of this literature by the presumed underlying mechanism of impact identifying at the outset the potential mediators and moderators of that impact; information gaps concerning specific points in the life course; the demands of policymakers. Relatively new to the canon of research about children's use of digital technologies is work on whether and how they impinge on children's mental health. Welfare officer work between 2003 and 2008 at my institution saw me leading conversations about whether and how contextually specific discourses of "stranger danger" and "inappropriate adult sites" were rational motivations for the institution to consider adopting great walls of filtering software and the student use policies and parental mailing home (in multiple languages) that would accompany this. There were a number of considerations and uncertainties: firstly, whether the legislative framework of the day enabled such surveillance of minors, and secondly and most relevant to this section of my thesis, there was very little empirically-based knowledge of the impact of such use on the well-being of children to guide these discussions. Whilst the quality data on children's use was time-stamped over a decade ago, there is some warrant for cautiously cashing some of it in. At the time of writing, the Office of Film and Literature Classification (OFLC) released an Internet Use Study (IUS) of 598 children aged 5 to 17 based on a nationwide, child-based survey. It reports a kick-up over recent years in children's access to computer devices compared with the 2007 and 2009 IUS surveys, with the two most ungeeky devices being mobile phones or tablets (before bedtime in half of the cases, after). The IUS was timed to inform new research on the development of a new classification office public awareness campaign of safe media use guidelines for parents.

*Scope and Significance of the Study*

This study is to explore the relationship between emerging technologies, secrecy, self-disclosure, and threat to the four developmental tasks. Finkelhor (1988) has identified developmental tasks of children, which include attachment to caregivers, mastery of the body, acquisition of education, and social integration including peer relations. To explore the relationship, this study will consider the effects of digital technology on these four dimensions. That is, we will explore the impact of secrecy and self-disclosure related to emerging technology on children and consider, also, the effects of increased surveillance on the extent to which children are meeting developmental milestones. The work of two scholars has informed the hypothesis that will be tested in the study.

This research is important for three groups of stakeholders. The first group affected by the relationship under study consists of children. Greater connection to emerging technology, and the consequences of increased secrecy and self-disclosure, have the potential to impact on key aspects of the lives of young people. A study of these issues with children as participants should illuminate how younger people react to these forms of threat. The conceptual understanding and empirical data generated by the project may be of use to medical and therapeutic institutions. This research can shed light on the character and extent of the relationship between emerging technology and child anxiety, and be of use in future development of practical tools. Finally, this project has implications for the future design, marketing, and application of new technologies.

## CHAPTER 1

# Understanding Childhood Anxiety

Childhood anxiety essentially refers to an intense, persistent, and irrational fear of everyday situations. Everyone experiences a degree of anxiety at some point, but it can be difficult to establish whether a child is experiencing normal worry or anxiety. Anxiety can make children more prone to experiencing negative emotions, such as anger or sadness, and they may become more prone to temper tantrums. Anxiety experienced by children tends to fall into three categories: 'risk aversion', 'anxiety disorders', and 'school-related anxiety'. Risk aversion is primarily concerned with children's refusal to try new things, from food to different activities and challenges, and will frequently encourage their parents to avoid exposing them to potentially difficult or new environments. Anxiety disorders are those that fall within the diagnosis guidelines established by the American Psychiatric Association. School-related anxiety in children is primarily rooted in concerns around bereavement, divorce, natural disasters, or terrorism. This type of anxiety experienced by children is not only exacerbated by digital media but played out through the media, too. Otherwise termed 'vicarious' anxiety, this type of anxiety is linked closely to the scope of this literature review and will therefore be the type of anxiety focused on here.

Vicarious experiences transmitted through digital media differ somewhat from other types of media-based experiences. Novel technologies are opening up an unprecedented blurring of the real and virtual domains, which sees the very nature of digital experiences differ somewhat from the so-called 'mass media'. One new development in psychological research—not only in relation to anxiety, but emotions more generally—entails examining the psychological responses associated with new developments in artificial or virtual experiences, or VR (virtual reality), experiences. Despite this very wide remit, many post-2000 digital technologies replicate elements of VR, making them increasingly relevant to psychological research. The digital technologies that allow children to most frequently experience others vicariously are social media, social networking sites (Facebook), vlogs (video blogs; YouTube), video streaming (Netflix), as well as digital games. Although these are most frequently associated with a passive reception of information about social others, they do incorporate a range of other features that allow a degree of two-way communication with the broadcasters, bloggers, gamers, and vloggers. Misuse and abuse of these communication features can also evoke changes in levels of anxiety, one might argue, but potential pathways from digital technology use to increases in children's vicarious anxiety induced by these alternative means are beyond our scope here.

## Definition and Types of Anxiety

Children experience worry and stress, just like adults do. One of the regular worries is school and grades. Technological advancements will offer new methods to detect and monitor childhood anxiety. Worries and stress are typical reactions to physical or emotional threats that individuals face. If left undetected, the impacts of suffering from mental health issues could be severe, and particularly for kids. Not only can untreated mental circumstances contribute to developing more destructive complications, but they can also cause difficulties in attention, peer relationships, and performance at school. Anxiety is a general term for many of these disorders.

There are several types of anxiety disorders, such as Generalized Anxiety Disorder (free floating), Social Anxiety (Social phobia), Specific Phobia, Separation Anxiety, Panic Disorder, Agoraphobia, and Obsessive-compulsive Disorder. Nevertheless, particular responses for anxiety problems embrace behavioral changes to cope with worry (i.e., withdrawal or avoidance), which reduces the chance of encountering doubt, or excessive distress about the potential experience. Users with anxiety problems perceive activities or experiences as hazardous when they are not or may overestimate the eventual negative result of a potential misfortune. Anxiety happens after a person is presented with stimuli that they or she has faced a mental image or memory of a former situation that resulted in an excessive degree of worry or loss. When the fear-inducing event is also current for the anxiety patient, the anxiety level would be understood as being out of the ordinary.

*Causes and Risk Factors*

Childhood anxiety is a serious public health issue. When left untreated, it often leads to a variety of negative physical and mental health outcomes, such as sleep disturbances, poor academic performance, increased risk of drug and alcohol abuse, and increased risk of psychiatric comorbidities, to name a few. It is well established that anxious children have problems functioning properly in both the home and school environments. Therefore, it is important to create a better understanding of the etiology of childhood anxiety in order to develop more effective treatments. There are many causes and risk factors that interact with each other to contribute to the development of anxiety in youth. It is therefore important to ask, "Is digital technology one of these factors that predispose children to developing anxiety?"

Smaller Amygdala - A smaller amygdala that has been observed in youths with anxiety disorders might be a result of the illness. A smaller amygdala has also been found in youths with autism, and while we are not arguing that having a smaller amygdala causes anxiety, there is some evidence to suggest that there is an inverse relationship between the size of the amygdala and anxiety in youths. However, further research in this domain is warranted. found that children with selective mutism have smaller amygdalae than children without SM. Children with smaller amygdalae also tended to have greater levels of social anxiety and behavioral problems. also found a smaller amygdala in socially anxious adolescents, and the effect was specific to social anxiety, which is of note. found that children with separation anxiety had larger amygdalae in comparison to other anxiety groups, while found no differences in amygdala volume in socially anxious youths when compared to non-anxious controls.

The interactions between parents and their children can also shape anxiety. studied the interaction of anxious mothers and their clinically anxious children and found that children initiated more contact and communication during a social problem-solving situation if a parent initiated more communication. More interestingly, the researchers found that more negative features of the interaction - as coded by an independent observer - had meaning tax for youths with social anxiety compared to control and anxious youths. Smaller Amygdala - A smaller amygdala that has been observed in youths with autism and also youths with anxiety disorders might be a result of the illness. However, the contrary may be posited that having a smaller amygdala is a risk factor for anxiety. Smaller amygdalae have been seen in socially anxious, physically abused, and institutionalized children, as well as in adults reminiscing about their childhoods and who had evidenced low childhood attachment security scores. Further research is warranted.

Deficits in connecting affect to autobiographical memories - A common theme in models of anxiety is the idea that individuals have emotional difficulties and differences. In May's model of separation anxiety and attachment difficulties, he posits that insecure dismissive individuals have less emotional reactivity, aversion to intimacy, higher rafts of gyn excreted when recalling stress narratives. and spies also posit that previously abused (highly anxious and depressed in this study) individuals had difficulty connecting affect to previously stored autobiographical narratives. Finally, social communication deficits are posited and have been studied as a primary genetic and endophenotypic feature of anxiety, somewhat linked to a socio-communicative model of autism and anxiety in youth. That is, in both conditions, deficits in communication and processing of socio-emotional stimuli are noted and may also be risk factors for the development of anxiety or autism or a combination of both conditions.

## CHAPTER 2

# The Digital Age: A New Frontier for Childhood Deve

The nature of childhood has undoubtedly been altered by the digital age. This essay now shifts towards discussing the ways in which the digitalized culture of today, with children in its throes, causes and is therefore linked to 21st-century childhood anxiety. Despite this, it has been suggested that the expansion of this age of digital technology comprises a new frontier, making available a space compatible with 'the rise of facts - quantifying, categorizing, measuring and comparing across all walks of life'. However, from a different perspective, this age might just as easily abstract itself from 'calendars and clocks, the body of flesh and blood, the earth, silence, and all other concrete particularities' to focus on the 'world of digital computation'. Herein lies a conundrum: digital analytics and the calculations they spin out are indeed the backdrop against which concepts about normalcy formation appear to be laced in the digital era. This era is also decisively intertwined with shifting youth, adult and parent perceptions around kids and tech. But the day-to-day psychological implications of growing up in such a digital age have yet to be deeply probed.

To begin to approach these implications is to enter into a theoretically diffuse field tested by a few pioneers. One of two pioneering themes, emerging as a point of rupture from the preceding section on not occasional anxiety, concerns the aporetic spaces of technology, subjectivity and illness-anxiety. Addressing this clustered dyad, Fukuyama tries to think through some of the knottier intersections of human nature and the anthropocentrism of tech. The influence of technology extends way back into our pre-enlightened past, where our 'most profound claim about technology in this realm is that life without it is a worse, more brutal life'. This hellishness, developed in Bush's time of the universal 'bomb', draws into its fold what Freud first called 'death-instinct'. A variation of this assurance appears with worry scenarios spun around the Adderall-riddled, next Bezos-genius syndrome. More, while the technological exists alongside our 'anger [as] post-human', it eventually refuses the empty 'outer shell' label some want to apply in 'shock value' terms to the digital self. More cautious than loud futurists chiseling themselves 'powerful images of apocalypse' stands Ovshinsky, precariously hinged around mental constraints rising 'if we make a wrong choice'.

*Evolution of Digital Technology*
The evolution of digital technology is a marvel to witness, from the first electronic computers to the internet and world wide web that permeates so much of the lives of global society. In a matter of decades, computers have become smaller, more powerful, faster, and less expensive. This technological evolution has brought personal computers, mobile phones, and other technology to the masses. With the advent of the internet, information is readily available and those connected have the ability to communicate with other likeminded or not-so-like-minded individuals the world over. Mechanisms like the internet, social media, use of cell phones and video

games have melded the lines of public and private spaces. The internet and related communications technology affect education, media, social communication, and psychologically much of what we do in life. In fact, they have changed the way individuals communicate, relate to one another and address anxiety.

It is crucial to understand how technology evolved, why it became so popular, and how it became such a ubiquitous form of communication throughout society, especially among families and children. Children in our society are growing up in a highly technological world where the prevalence of technology, including internet, social media, and personal devices, is ever increasing. As a result of this exposure, children are adopting the use of these devices faster than ever before. In the United States, 96% of children between the ages of 3-18 have access to some technological device and 88% of their schools use computers in the classroom. This figure is not unique to the United States; it is similar in other countries and continents as well. Also, in 2015, 24% of the people living in developing countries had access to the internet; 10% increase from the year before.

*Benefits and Risks of Digital Technology for Children*

Many children develop competence in using digital technology faster than their parents or teachers. They can use digital technology to find information, acquire knowledge of the world, and contact and communicate with others. They appear to thrive on the ability to access numerous sources of information simultaneously and to concentrate on more than one task. Exposing a child to digital technology from an early age may also develop interventions to bring extra enjoyment to daily life. Moreover, it may develop hand-eye coordination skills, and attention and vision may be improved. Technology employed such as tablets, smartphones, or even computers can also significantly improve social networking and voice recognition for children, especially for those with hearing differences or problems with speech.

However, despite all the benefits the digital technology will bring to a child, there are also risks. Children who spend long periods online will take more chances. This is because they are engrossed and they ignore dangers. The time spent in child management and social activities will eventually decrease. The child picks which websites are available and, in turn, what they view and access. When spent, digital technology will then lead to less energy and less sleep, which contributes to mental and emotional disorders such as stress or depression. It may also be that intense feelings of anxiety are caused by anxiety that can result in intense reactions. Nevertheless, because the risks may vary from one child to another, it is important to consider a child's life when it comes to the use of digital resources.

# CHAPTER 3

# The Intersection of Digital Technology and Childho

In recent years, childhood anxiety has become a booming field of exploration. However, research is often situated within individualistic and pathologizing paradigms that center symptoms and fail to consider the social climate in which anxiety arises, as well as the myriad ways that childhood can contribute to the etiology and maintenance of anxiety. Additionally, the kind of external events children are anxious about – such as pandemics and school shootings – hardly ever gets discussed, creating a myopia and lack of concreteness to our understandings of anxiety. In addition to building on this school, there is a wealth of thinking about how various entities of childhood, including adults and nonhumans, may play a role in creating and maintaining anxiety.

One key area needing further exploration is the ways that digital technologies may contribute to anxiety in childhood. Amidst the proliferation of digital tech, research indicates that the time spent on such screens is positively correlated with depression and anxiety. In response, a wariness of excessive screen time, and a hope that decreased screen time will lessen symptoms of anxiety, has become widespread. However, I argue that this angle of analysis is overly simplistic. In this section, I flatten the several ways that digital tech can impact, activate, or exacerbate anxiety.

*Screen Time and Mental Health*

Introducing the statistics makes it clear that the impact of technology on childhood in the UK has reached endemic proportions. More than half of all five to 16-year-olds have a social media profile (ONS, 2021), with 3 to 4-year-olds averaging 8 hours and 18 minutes screen time per day (OfCom, 2021). Further questioning of this topic's importance brings into play the question of child health crises, which seep from the heart of the casual internet user. Highlighting an increasingly anxious generation seems to suggest that there is an overall increase in childhood anxiety that impacts even the most confident and resilient of children. Between 17 June 2019 and 21 June 2021, 12 to 16-year-old girls were 53% more likely to be diagnosed with anxiety than boys (NHS, Mental Health of Children and Young People, 2021), although they continue to report feeling more anxious across the board as one-in-three 16-year-olds having undergone an anxiety disorder in secondary school (The Department for Education, 2021).

Without the support of comprehensive psychological data, and considering the broader spread of poor mental health, it would be disingenuous to conclude that societal changes previously increasingly relegated to schools have not spilled over into isolation-prone home learning households. Examinations of touch screen/digital technologies and their impact on childhood mental health indicate a potential increased prevalence of anxiety. MacKillop (2018) shows that screen time use is reciprocally linked to mental health issues, as child users report less happy feelings and suffer from increased internalizing factors of predominantly social anxiety and depressive states. Wolf and Sumner (2020) continue this conversation by undermining child use of devices as merely "screen time," and instead focusing on power and status. Their research critically explores ethical technological use in the context of social identity, emphasizing the fact that screen time "tears children from the healthy toys of life" and isolates children to the interior of the home (Wolf & Sumner, 2020). Continuing this sentiment, Gunasekera & Hopkin (2019) discuss the effect of accelerated developmental and psychological attachment (also echoed by Reid-Chung today) between children and digital devices, stating that to separate this duo would "stimulate high levels of anxiety in their mother."

*Social Media and Peer Relationships*

The impact of digital technology on the peer relationships of children has often been discussed in the media. Turning to social media, some authors have detailed the processes by which this engagement affects the child. Some discussions focus on the highly constructed nature of selfies and photos in which children present themselves in a way they believe will attract likes from their friends. This was presented in a negative light and was seen as a risky way of children regulating their feelings of safety and connection. Programming a social reward for presenting oneself in one way was called 'manipulation'.

While the replication of peer exclusion that can occur away from the screen was noted, positive interpretations of social media's impact on friendships are scarce in British media. When considered as another way to keep in touch with those we know, social media was noted positively. The negatives of young people's use of social media, which has been identified in the media, carries some implications for children's mental health. Teenagers worrying over the potential loss of connection with their friends from a break in the use of screen technology shows that the nature of online social life is having the effect of increasing anxiety. Further studies should directly investigate the contribution that online forms of communication are making to the reported increase in adolescents' anxiety to establish the magnitude of the effect. A preliminary hypothesis is that its impact is likely to be relatively small. Many of the social rules that seem derogatory when applied to online communications are frequently ignored in face-to-face conversations. Plenty of time is also spent by many digital natives away from their screens.

**CHAPTER 4**

# Parenting in the Digital Age

It is beyond argument that the digital world can have potentially negative impacts on childhood mental health. Our advice to parents is not to abandon digital parenting—it is inevitable in the 21st century and can offer many educational opportunities—but to adopt strategies that reflect the research evidence. Downplaying internet and social media fears at the expense of providing accurate and evidence-based advice is not helpful for parents. Increasingly, it is becoming more difficult to shelter children from digital technology and many parents are starting to wake up to this reality. Strategies parents mention include making sure all digital devices are out of the bedroom so that the child cannot access them freely at night, encouraging their child to talk about what they do online and make sure they understand the risks and are prepared to manage these, just as they are in daily life, and having family discussions about safe and appropriate use of the internet.

Children as young as four now have their own social media profile pages and there is a trend in unsupervised use, according to parents, of by tod's financially strapped schools offering the use of tablets and iPods to help children with learning. Furthermore, gaming apps are becoming increasingly popular with children as young as three to five, something which app developers refer to as a sort of trend where children are getting more involved in interactive and educational game apps. Use is increasing every year with new models, greater access, and parental purchasing power. Thus, the digital revolution is all pervasive; in a study of 1000 families, four years after Christmas one in five homes were now using digital tablets on a daily basis, two children took these tablets to bed, and over half used them on the long car ride to the store. It is now not uncommon to see digital tablets, smartphones, and other devices being used to help with 'settling' children in cafes and restaurants. Have tablets and smartphones now become a replacement for social engagement, reading, and family time (talk, sing, play with me)? With the digital revolution, children face many new risks in the modern age of technology. Screen exposure to digital media is quite seductive and for some kids can become an obsessive time-draining experience—overuse can have potential effects on family relationships as kids may opt to engage in solitary time in a digitized world rather than join their parents.

*Challenges and Strategies for Parents*

Parents nowadays encounter various challenges in the digital information age. They hold diverse views on children's internet devices, media exposure, and mobile devices. While the internet can improve children's learning in terms of digital resilience and screen-time exposure, this can cause anxiety and other psychiatric symptoms. The increase in parental concern is associated with searching "anxiety in children" as related to the Covid-19 pandemic. The internet helps us to confront, manage, cope, and prevent childhood anxiety during the digital revolution. A search of the literature and current affairs was conducted regarding internet, digital technology, and child/adolescent cybersickness on-related childhood anxiety. The databases were systematically searched on the topic, and the results are presented in this review.

For parents, digital technology in this digital era can help children cope with the fluency of digital problems themselves to regulate childhood anxiety in cybersickness. Because cybersickness has been neglected, especially among children, the parents need the theoretical foundation for digital navigation. This paper concludes by providing resources and practical strategies for parents and professionals in digital cybersickness to overcome childhood anxiety. Strategies and key principles for parents, caregivers, and professionals to assuage the negative impact of the digital revolution on childhood anxiety should include but not be exclusive to balancing screen time with outdoor engagement. Engaging children with different eye levels and adjusting the screen angle can engage the parasympathetic and sympathetic nervous systems in a balanced manner. It can decrease the cortisol level of anxiety in the brain.

## CHAPTER 5

# Schools and Mental Health Support

Both the Department for Education and Public Health England have recognized the importance of school in the well-being of children, promoting prevention and early intervention for social, emotional, and mental health. In 2017, schools were given legal responsibility for addressing the emotional well-being of their students. The government has outlined guidance for schools, stipulating an expectation that Children and Young People's Mental Health (CYPMH) Support Teams liaise with schools to provide support for children with emerging mental health issues earlier. This early support is funded by the money allocated to CYP mental health detention. 'Early help' makes more sense than leaving it to get bad and the child needing lengthy interventions down the line. The guidance documents do not make explicit how digital technology could cause harm to children's and young people's mental health, but we know.

There are a few things educational institutions can do to help combat the issues caused by technology to very young children. In addition to guidance for parents, their children and young people, the government's 'Teaching Online Safety in Schools' document cites strategies to promote the use of technology in a positive manner. One of the strategies is to raise awareness that it is also normal to feel overwhelmed because of the digital environment and instead of just teaching about the devices themselves, a cumulative cross-curricular approach could be used to further help equip children to handle the digital environment. Governor and governor training also form part of promoting a Healthy School, creating an environment and opportunities for physical, social, emotional, and physical well-being. Full Ofsted inspections can take place every 5 years, the expectations for which are outlined in the Inspection Handbook. Favorable grades are given for those schools providing proactive and quality PSHE lessons for the students, which will include aspects of life online, DFLA, mental health, and e-safety.

*The Role of Schools in Addressing Childhood Anxiety*

With increasing numbers of children suffering from mental health conditions, there is a growing interest in schools as sites for prevention and early intervention. The number of initiatives and resources that focus on supporting children's social, emotional, and mental health has seen a significant increase, fueled in part by the data from the Foundations for Life report and other data on the benefits of good emotional wellbeing. This increase is also a likely reaction to the profound social and technological changes that have taken place over recent years. Along with the wider social context, the range and types of issues that schools may have to confront have changed. Various media reports have postulated links between new forms of technology use and an increase in mental health conditions such as anxiety and depression. A study by NHS Digital adds to this by finding that among 5-19-year-olds, emotional disorders have become more common since 2009 (11%). For children aged 5-15, their own experiences include the ability to find information and keep in touch easily as a result of remedial technology that many use (organic). Issues which result from the conscious and potentially harmful side of technology are indicated by one in five reporting they have been the subject of bullying (20%) in some form or another.

At school, the shift to the digital age is possibly felt most acutely in the classroom. Schools have had to adapt children's formal learning experiences to a rapidly changing outside world. The traditional classroom technologies, such as electronic whiteboards, are supplemented with a plethora of web-based teaching tools, homework submission sites, information platforms for parents. At the same time, schools have had to get to grips with the psycho-educational landscape in which many pupils are active users of a variety of devices, social media platforms, and associated socializing and learning opportunities. In terms of physical equipment, for older children, the majority (87%) report that they have three or more digital devices of their own. This is in addition to equipment that is shared with family members. Beyond personal ownership of digital devices, the children at schools are educated with are relatively cheap and accessible in the age of the digital bartering economy. While schools must be equipping children for the digital age, they still face having to confront the potential mental health issues of such a mediated experience. Knowing the difference between a child who is negotiating friendships and might need a cuddle because their heart is sore and a child who is exhibiting a diagnosable mental health condition is part of everyday practice for school staff. It is therefore valuable to understand where technology use might fit in with a current school-based anti-anxiety framework. This current primary role that schools can play has been placed in the context of the school's wider work on the mental health and well-being of pupils.

## CHAPTER 6

# Future Directions for Research and Policy

This conceptual paper focuses on recent research and practice addressing digital technology and childhood anxiety. In this light, we now envisage future developments in this burgeoning field. We begin by considering the most important directions for research, seeking to generate benefits for young people while attending to both individual needs and broader social issues. We then set out policy questions that need to be addressed in order to support greater well-being while making the most of advances in technology. We recognize the role digital technologies have played in supporting learning and sociality for many young people during the COVID-19 pandemic, but also the disparities in accessibility that have emerged during this time. We identify four key themes: augmenting the evidence base, addressing both needs and strengths and targeting those who need it most, encouraging engagement, and digital citizenship and online safety.

It is likely that research focusing on digital technologies and childhood anxiety will increasingly converge on a small number of areas. Those exploring mental health impacts may adopt more fine-grained research designs than in the past, perhaps implementing stepped care with increasing intensity. This increasingly turns to the research on practice and away from randomized controlled trials reviewing if digital treatments work 'at all' and emphasizes the more pertinent research question of 'do they work compared to what?'. Furthermore, within-person trials are likely to increase in popularity, particularly in relation to the self-regulation model of anxiety. Such research designs would inform both the practice elements of the seemingly low-intensity digital interventions and may begin to confirm specific guidance given in Nice about personalized digital interventions and the optimal person symptom, cognitive, and learning style characteristics for engaging. The use of such methods may be facilitated by increased access to digital data through, for instance, online learning sites. The use of automated speech analysis is an example of one method that could be combined with within-person trials to predict change in anxiety symptoms over time from both children and parent reports on automatic scoring of parent interactions with children. We may also see an increase in lab-based studies of the effects of digital technologies on change variables, for instance, attentional bias to threat, interpretation biases, or treatment-enhancing variables such as trust. This will likely see the boundaries between 'online' and 'offline' studies reducing and methods and results synthesizing with the wider learning and attention bias literatures.

*Emerging Trends and Technologies*

Emerging trends and technologies. Key trends you might find in the next few years that could impact this area: As the technology that we have access to evolves at an ever-increasing pace, it is suggested here that our strategies for supporting young people should also evolve. This essay has explored the relationship between digital technology and childhood anxiety, outlining what is currently known about what can be a significant stressor for young people. Happily, what we do know suggests that there are actions that can be taken to support young people. Making recommendations for interventions can be tricky when there is little accessible research backing up those options. However, the rich seam of existing research stating clearly what adults and young people want from mental health services (in which digital technology ranks high) gives us a jumping-off point for using some of the digital interventions that are out there for young people.

This could be an approach for further research and some investment, and so better explored in Years 3-5. I submit that this is a rich area for future work because of the rapidly-evolving technology landscape. We can identify a few potential foci for further work now. Therefore, from Year 3 onwards, a combination of quantitative and qualitative work around those recommendations will be helpful. For example: Surveys of adults and young people asking them about current barriers to intervention use. An equal scope would be to survey the providers of psychological interventions for young people, in order to find out whether they are currently able to offer digitally-based interventions; and if not, why not. Quantitative work with adults and young people exploring their digital mental health/digital mental health literacy, building out the insight from the scoping diagram to find out what platforms and apps are currently being used. This can and should be viewed as a way to monitor what children and parents are currently accessing and their perceptions of this range.

# CHAPTER 7

# Conclusion

The coming conclusion is aimed at summarizing the insights generated throughout the essay regarding the impact of digital technology on childhood anxiety. The conclusion draws upon the findings and discusses the importance of the evidence reviewed for practice, policy, and services with young people. Finally, the conclusion will end with exploring the limitations of the body of work reviewed and where the future direction of research may lie.

The essay has provided evidence that the way in which digital technology is used can be both a risk and a protective factor in relation to the experience of childhood anxiety. Digital technologies place a high demand on the developing self-regulation skills of young people. Online external pressures, such as cyberbullying, and pressures to work on online school lessons exacerbate this. The FGC children and young people participating in the study reported some relief in mental intrusion due to the need for hyper-vigilance being curtailed during lockdown. However, some new anxiety presented due to a lack of contact with the outside world. Findings show that action around future traditional evidence gathering and risk assessment may be methodologically flawed. There is a need for a more direct and ethical use of listening to those with lived experience, particularly our children and young people, in order to ensure that we are establishing outcomes that are more meaningful and responsive to threats that they perceive. These findings replicate some suggestions made in the vast research conducted during and after WW2 on listening to children during times of conflict. There are practical implications in relation to technology, legal, policy, and procedural implications. The internet and remote learning have played a key role in perpetrating threats alerted to in this rapid consultation.

Further investigation is needed surrounding the psychological impact digital technology has on children during child protection processes. The western literature is voluminous; however, no work seems to have been published on the subject as it relates to child protection: there must be some. More qualitative research is required in relation to technology and the voices of all stakeholders within the child protection experience. Can we make any conclusive arguments on the matter? No. All we can do is draw ideas on the matter based on the Bible of the FGC model. We can then have a genuine and informed debate that could pave a way forward as we further aim to understand the factors, incidentals of impact, and best legal pathways on the developing brain of children, both good and bad. In other words, all we can do is think. Our paper has inserted academics into the debate on the fallacies of routine evidence and given a voice to a reluctant and marginalized group. Our work is satisfied that the questions stemming from both academic and public debate are worthy of publication and should be inserted into general medical journals.

*Summary of Key Findings*

Key findings: The results begin by considering young people's use of digital technologies. Despite ongoing concerns about possible negative effects on children's and young people's mental health or anxiety, there are consistent statistical trends across both qualitative and quantitative research findings suggesting little difference in most respects between those young people who use digital technologies and those who do not. Discrepancies in the findings are most notable in the domain of mental health. It is clear that a range of protective factors helps young people manage in an environment where there is much concern about potential risks. These include relational support and a mediated experience of the online world. Despite a commercial market that often promotes many of the qualities of digital life that could be damaging for overall wellbeing, young people tend to not seek commercial support - or that proffered by government, formal industry or international regulators. Instead, they use their interpersonal worlds for support.

There is a gap in the literature that specifically seeks to understand the mental health consequences of digital technologies. There are few empirical studies, or studies based on the unsolicited experiences of young people, which try to definitively explore what role digital technologies play in unwellness or mental morbidity. Here, it is young people's descriptions of their acute experiences of digital technologies that yield initial suggestions about disaffection, depression, or anxiety. Participants describe perceptions of digital experiences being 'risky' to their self-concept - that others are positioned as people like them with whom others can readily compare. There are other suggestions made in the data that have the potential for evoking anxiety: concerns about being out of the social 'loop' and about losing time to consumption. Participants reflect on their own anxieties and suggest that experiences are widespread: digital opportunity might place a demand on them or on their professional future or abilities. They also pose that by using digital technologies they might have a normal level of alertness about their place or status, but at the extremes (and including bipolar disorder) mental ill-health may make people more alert to socio-economic issues that create widespread disaffection.

*Implications for Practice and Policy*

The results suggest that, given the uncertainties in this field, decisions about how to guide or help children with managing their digital lives should be pragmatic and should aim to address the full range of determinants of anxiety and mental health rather than focusing entirely on digital technology. This includes paying close attention to the broader psychological context, such as family issues, the quality of peer relationships, and wider processes of socialisation. However, included below are some distilled implications specifically in relation to policy and practice.

Substance suggests that it may not be wise or useful to make sweeping recommendations about which activities children should and should not do in relation to screen and internet use. Practitioners should work with children and parents to identify individual situations where digital technology may be exacerbating anxiety and to provide tools to help manage anxiety in these cases. Practitioners should aim to equip children and parents with requisite knowledge to improve their digital literacy. Practitioners should be included in any research or implementation of interventions in the digital world to ensure feedback and learning can be integrated into approaches as it becomes apparent. Policy makers and developers of apps or interventions targeted at children should have input from children and practitioners to ensure approaches designed to reduce anxiety among children are appropriate and sensitive to different population groups. Policy makers should be cautious about investing public money into practice in belief that it will reduce childhood anxiety in the absence of evidence in the academic literature.

www.ingramcontent.com/pod-product-compliance
Lightning Source LLC
LaVergne TN
LVHW042252070526
838201LV00104B/296